Keto Bread

50 Quick & Easy Low-Carb Ketogenic Recipes Including Delicious Breads, Bagels, Muffins, Cakes & More!

Claire Stapleton

© Copyright 2019 by Cascade Publishing

All rights reserved.

It is not legal to reproduce, duplicate, or transmit any part of this document in either electronic means or in printed format. Recording of this publication is strictly prohibited.

CONTENTS

Introduction 1
Baking Tips 2
    Low Carb Flours 7
    Low Carb Sweeteners 9
Macadamia Nut Loaf 10
Cauliflower Tortillas 12
Blueberry Muffins 14
Chocolate and Zucchini Bread 16
French Crepes 18
Olive, Feta and Red Pepper Mini Muffins 20
Tomato Pesto Tart with Cauliflower Crust 22
Dark Chocolate and Sea Salt Cookies 25
Garlic and Cheese Crackers 27
Rosemary and Sea Salt Focaccia 29
Mojito Cupcakes 32
Rosemary Cheddar Cornbread 35
Jalapeno Popper Pittas 37
Chocolate Donuts 39
Rye Bread 41
Cauliflower Breadsticks 43
Zucchini Pizza 45
Chocolate and Peanut Butter Protein Balls 47
Cloud Bread 49
Lavender Shortbread 51
Pepperoni Pizza Quiche 53
Squid Ink Rolls 55
Cardamom, Rose and Pistachio Scones 57
Pumpkin Pie 59

Salted Caramel Apple Tart 62

Cheese and Pesto Pinwheels 65

Gingerbread Men 68

Sundried Tomato Bread 70

Rainbow Cinnamon Rolls 72

Gruyère, Onion and Thyme Tear & Share 75

Coffee Cake 77

Cheese, Garlic and Red Pesto Twists 79

Poppy Seed Bagels 81

Chocolate Pistachio Shortbread 83

Chocolate Orange Cake Pops 85

Red Velvet Pancakes 87

Easy Crumpets 89

Banana and Chocolate Bread 91

Beetroot Brownies 93

Parmesan Croutons 95

Avocado Chocolate Cake 97

Courgette, Lemon & Mascarpone Cupcakes 100

Sourdough 102

Peanut Butter Cookies 104

Pretzels 106

Coconut Macaroons 108

Cumin Naan 110

Carrot Cake Cookies 112

Chocolate Pizza 114

Spicy Cheese Taco Shells 117

Conclusion 119

Introduction

There are many reasons why you may have decided to follow a keto diet. It could be for weight loss, an intolerance, or to prevent a future illness which is beginning to worry you. Despite what you might think, there's not one type of person who follows a keto diet and there's not one set menu, either. We hope this *'Keto Bread'* recipe book allows you to experiment with some of the foods which were once written on your 'not to eat' list. In fact, we implore you to specifically choose the foods you have once avoided.

However, rather than munching away on these foods without a second thought, try eating mindfully. Every ingredient has been carefully selected to taste delicious, *and* make you feel good. We believe that every day can be a treat, every meal should bring you happiness, and your health does not need to be compromised.

We have never been very good at following the rules, and we don't think you should be either. So have fun, experiment and change up each and every recipe to fit the needs of you and your family! We have worked out the nutritional contents of each bake so that you can concentrate on the baking, and eating without concern.

Baking Tips

Ever wonder how some people get perfect results time after time while your bakes come out looking worse for wear? Follow our expert advice to guarantee brilliant bakes with every recipe.

Let all liquids get to room temperature

This should be the first step for all baking, and cannot be skipped in keto recipes. Ingredients with different temperatures have a hard time binding, which means you could end up with a lumpy or split batter.

Don't be stingy with baking powder

You'll notice baking power featuring more heavily in keto recipes than you might be used to, but fear not, this just helps alternative flours rise and creates light and airy bakes. You should never be able to taste the extra!

Keto 'milks'

Regular milk is not ideal for a keto diet as it's high in sugar and carbs. Luckily, there are many great alternatives that you can do a direct swap with. We love almond, coconut and flax milk!

Flax eggs

Eggs and keto are very good friends, however, you'll notice some of the keto recipes you come across will mention flax eggs - a water and flax mixture which in many recipes can take on the qualities of an egg. This is because many people who follow a keto diet also choose to follow other diets simultaneously, like dairy-free. Flax eggs are also great for people with egg allergies.

1 Tbsp of ground Flax seeds + 3 Tbsp water + 15 minutes in the fridge to thicken = one flax egg

Not all flours are created equally

Although most of your favorite recipes can be 'ketofied' with a little creativity, you cannot directly swap a grain flour for an alternative, or even a coconut flour for almond, as they're all totally unique, weigh differently and hold different properties. Always double check online for the correct conversion before swapping out flours.

With fewer ingredients to hide behind, go for the best quality you can afford.

Most of the baked goods we buy from the supermarket have an incredibly long and unpronounceable ingredients list containing vast amounts of salt and sugar, which mask the low quality and artificial ingredients found lower down the never-ending list. You'll be able to taste many if not all of the few ingredients in your home baking so make them count and go for organic where possible.

All good bakes begin with a sift.

The importance of sifting flour is no different in keto recipes than it is in any other baking, and is essential for light and fluffy, none lumpy results. When sieving almond flour you may find that a lot is wasted which doesn't go through the holes, so instead of using a regular sieve, we recommend blending it in a food processor until fine, as always, being careful not to over blend.

How to tell when your bake is, baked

Not all ovens are equal. What's 350F in my oven may be less in yours, and as well as thickness in baking pans, differences in ingredients and a multitude of other reasons, the suggested cooking time can only ever be taken as a suggestion. So spend some time with your oven and don't be afraid to have a peep inside to check everything is going on okay. You can always bake your item for longer, but once your item has dried out or burned, then there's really no going back. Try and learn what your '350F' is and make notes on the recipes you frequent so you don't forget. This goes for microwaves and even hob plates, too.

When baking any types of sponge

Skewer, toothpick, knife… whatever your weapon of choice may be, the more baking you do the more reliant you'll be on this unassuming object. Once you have reached the desired color and rise of your sponge it's time to carefully insert your skewer into the center of your bake and if it comes out clean you should be done. If there's residue then you need another five minutes before you try again.

The smaller the instrument you choose, the less you'll interrupt the baking process. So avoid forks or anything too thick.

This technique does not work for gooey, fudgy recipes and you'll be waiting a very long time to see a clean skewer come out of a tray of brownies!

When baking muffins or cupcakes

Just in case the heat in your oven isn't evenly distributed, choose one in the center and either side of the tray to test.

When baking bread

Once you have tried the above skewer trick, check the color. The type of bread you're baking will determine the color you desire, however, with most varieties you should aim for golden brown.

Once this box has been ticked and you're tempted to take it out to cool, flip it around and gently tap the base. If you have a hollow sound then your bread will be light and baked, if not, then your bread will still be dense and doughy inside and needs at least another five minutes.

When baking cookies

If your cookie looks finished when you take it out of the oven, you got to it at least five minutes too late. This won't affect the taste too much, but you will have a hard and brittle cookie and a potential work out for your teeth. Fear not though, over baked cookies often soften in a sealed cookie jar after a day or two, and if it's really beyond repair then they make great cheesecake bases crumbled up and mixed with butter.

You might think of baking as a peaceful and relaxing hobby but when it comes to checking your bakes, you need to act fast! The longer the oven door is open, cold air is pouring in, and it takes very little time for the temperature to change. Try not to open the oven until you are fairly certain your bake is finished, this way the basic structure will be formed and you are less likely to suffer sinking, uneven rises or air bubbles.

If you notice a bake cooking too quickly (it may have risen very high, very fast or started to get dark on top whilst the middle is still uncooked) then lower the oven temperature and create an umbrella of aluminum foil above it to stop it darkening any further on top.

Ingredients

This is the most important and crucial part. It's thanks to ingredients like these which make your favorite sweet and savory snacks possible while on a Ketogenic diet.

Low Carb Flours

There are lots more fantastic flour alternatives available! Below are some of our favorites.

Coconut Flour

A by-product of coconut milk, this grain and gluten-free flour is made from powdered coconut flesh so a faint coconut flavor may be present in you bake. An especially great choice for nut-free bakers. It's popular in both sweet and savory recipes and works well for thickening soups and sauces, binding burgers and coating wet or sticky ingredients.

Almond Flour / Meal / Ground almonds

A readily available, flavorsome and gluten-free flour alternative made from blanched, ground almonds.

Ground Flax / Flax Meal

Flax seeds are highly recommended for their health benefits. These little seeds are packed with healthy fats, minerals and vitamins, and very few calories. Top tip: they become much easier to digest when ground rather than whole.

Psyllium Husk

A healthy fiber made from the husks of the Plantago ovata seeds, and highly popular for weight loss.

Low Carb Sweeteners

There's many great alternatives to table sugar but here are some of our favorites.

Stevia

Stevia is a very popular sweetener due to the variety of forms it comes in. From liquid drops to granulated or even as a powder - not to mention the many different flavor options available.

Erythritol

A low-calorie sugar alcohol with 70% of the sweetness of cane sugar.

Monk Fruit Sweetener

Monk fruit is a much sweeter alternative to sugar so you don't need to add a lot to your recipes. It's 100% natural and has a glycemic index of 0 so you don't get any of the spikes in your blood pressure which sugar causes.

Xylitol

A popular sugar alcohol and refined sweetener with a very low glycemic index and low calories deriving from tree fiber.

Macadamia Nut Loaf

This fluffy macadamia bread is wrapped in a delicious, grain-free crust - extremely addictive and surprisingly healthy! Perfect straight out of the oven or toasted the next day, this versatile loaf was made for creamy peanut butter and rainy afternoons.

Serves: 10 slices

Ingredients

- 1 cup macadamia nuts
- 5 large eggs
- ¼ cup coconut flour
- 1 tsp sea salt
- ½ tsp baking powder
- ½ Tbsp apple cider vinegar
- 2 Tbsp pumpkin seeds

Method

1. Preheat the oven to 350F and prepare an 8x4 loaf pan.
2. Create a nut flour by pouring the macadamia nuts in a food processor and blending until fine.
3. Whilst blending, add each egg until you reach a

smooth consistency.

4. Mix in the coconut flour, sea salt, and apple cider vinegar until combined.
5. Fill the loaf pan ¾ full and sprinkle with pumpkin seeds.
6. Bake for 30-40 minutes, until golden or a skewer comes out clean.
7. Allow to cool for 20 minutes (if you can wait), slice into 10 pieces and serve!

Nutrition per serving

Calories: 155

- **Total Fat** 13.8g
- Saturated Fat 2.8g
- **Cholesterol** 93mg
- **Sodium** 223mg
- **Total Carbohydrate** 4.8g
- Dietary Fiber 2.6g
- Total Sugars 0.8g
- **Protein** 5.1g

Cauliflower Tortillas

These healthy and versatile tortillas make replacement taco shells, filling breakfasts or an easy and delicious snack. Mix up the seasoning, add a little heat or just enjoy as they are for a crowd-pleasing and comforting take on a Mexican classic.

Serves: 4

Ingredients

- ¾ large head cauliflower (or two cups riced)
- 2 large eggs
- ¼ cup chopped fresh cilantro
- ½ medium lime (juiced and zested)
- 4 cloves of garlic (peeled and crushed)
- Sea salt and cracked black pepper, to taste

Method

1. Preheat the oven to 375F and prepare a baking tray.
2. Cut the cauliflower into 1cm pieces, and blend in a food processor until you achieve a grain-like consistency.
3. Lightly fry the crushed garlic until soft.

4. Microwave the cauliflower for 2 minutes, then stir and repeat. Once cooled slightly, place the cauliflower in a fine cloth and squeeze out as much liquid as you can and add the cauliflower to a dry, medium-sized bowl.
5. Mix in the remaining ingredients until combined.
6. Roll out 6 even balls with your hands and press them down them on the lined tray, creating flat tortillas shapes.
7. Bake for 10 minutes, carefully flipping each tortilla and returning to the oven for an additional 5 to 7 minutes.
8. Brown each tortilla for 1 to 2 minutes on each side in a medium heated skillet and enjoy!

Nutrition per serving

Calories: 82

- **Total Fat** 2.7g
- Saturated Fat 0.8g
- **Cholesterol** 93mg
- **Sodium** 83mg
- **Total Carbohydrate** 10.5g
- Dietary Fiber 4.3g
- Total Sugars 4.2g

Protein 6.5g

Blueberry Muffins

These delicious blueberry muffins are all the joy of a Sunday morning treat but healthy enough to have them every day of the week and believe us, you will do!

Serves: 12

Ingredients

- 2 ½ cup blanched almond flour
- ½ cup erythritol
- 1 ½ tsp gluten-free baking powder
- ¼ tsp sea salt
- ⅓ cup coconut oil (measured solid, then melted)
- ⅓ cup unsweetened almond milk
- 3 large eggs
- ½ tsp vanilla extract
- ¾ cup blueberries

Method

1. Preheat the oven to 350F and prepare a muffin pan.
2. In a large bowl, stir together the almond flour, erythritol, baking powder, and sea salt

3. Mix in the wet ingredients and carefully add the blueberries.
4. Spoon the batter evenly into the muffin cases.
5. Bake for 20-25 minutes, until golden and a skewer comes out clean.
6. Leave to cool before removing from the pan and enjoy!

Nutrition per serving

Calories: 113

- Total Fat 10.2g
- Saturated Fat 5.9g
- Cholesterol 47mg
- Sodium 162mg
- Total Carbohydrate 2.9g
- Dietary Fiber 0.9g
- Total Sugars 1g
- Protein 2.9g

Chocolate and Zucchini Bread

This moist and moreish loaf is an unlikely combination of green power and dark chocolate but the result is like nothing else!

Serves: 12

Ingredients

- ½ cup coconut flour
- ½ cup unsweetened cocoa powder
- ½ cup Splenda sweetener
- 1 tsp baking soda
- 1 tsp gluten-free baking powder
- ¼ tsp salt
- ¼ cup coconut oil (melted)
- 4 large eggs
- 1 tsp vanilla
- 2 cups zucchini (grated)
- ½ cup dark chocolate chips

Method

1. Preheat the oven to 350F and prepare a 9X5 loaf pan.
2. In a large bowl combine the dry ingredients.

3. Mix in the eggs, coconut oil, and vanilla until well combined.

4. Add the grated zucchini and dark chocolate chips.

5. Pour the mixture into the pan and bake for 45-55 minutes or until a skewer comes out clean.

6. Remove from oven and cool completely before serving!

Nutrition per serving

Calories: 98

- Total Fat 5.8g
- Saturated Fat 2.7g
- Cholesterol 62mg
- Sodium 262mg
- Total Carbohydrate 16.2g
- Dietary Fiber 6.8g
- Total Sugars 3.2g
- Protein 4.1g

French Crepes

Transport yourself to a chic and cozy cafe in Paris with these moreish and light pancakes. This French specialty is temptingly quick and simple to create but just as delicious as the real thing.

Serves: 4

Ingredients

Crepes

- 8 eggs
- 2 cups heavy whipping cream
- ½ cups water
- ¼ tsp salt
- 2 tsp ground psyllium husk powder
- 4 Tbsp coconut oil

Optional

- 1 cups whipped coconut cream
- 1 cups fresh berries
- Powdered stevia to taste

Method

1. Use a hand mixer to combine eggs, cream, water, and salt.

2. Slowly mix in the psyllium husk until you achieve a smooth batter and rest for 15 minutes.

3. Lightly fry a small amount of coconut oil in your frying pan at medium heat before pouring in the batter. Fry the crepes on each side but let it get 90% dry before flipping to avoid sticking.

4. Serve with whipped coconut cream and fresh berries for the perfect, Parisian treat!

Nutrition per serving

Calories: 461

- Total Fat 44.7g
- Saturated Fat 28.3g
- Cholesterol 410mg
- Sodium 294mg
- Total Carbohydrate 2.4g
- Dietary Fiber 0g
- Total Sugars 0.8g
- Protein 12.7g

Olive, Feta and Red Pepper Mini Muffins

These fluffy and flavorsome mini muffins are one bite wonders - as quick and easy to make as they are to eat. Try substituting the vegetables for your family favorites for a versatile and filling breakfast.

Serves: 12 Mini muffins

Ingredients

- 1 ½ fresh spinach
- olive oil
- 4 eggs
- ¼ cup water
- 1 Tbsp dried oregano
- ¼ pinch of sea salt
- ¼ pinch of black pepper
- ¼ cup butter (melted and unsalted)
- ⅓ cup coconut flour
- ¼ tsp baking soda
- ¼ cup parmesan cheese
- ¼ cup feta cheese (cubed)
- ¼ cup black olives (chopped finely)
- ½ cup red peppers (chopped finely)

Method

1. Preheat the oven to 400F degrees and prepare a pan with 16 mini muffin cups.
2. Fry the spinach in olive oil until wilted and set aside.
3. Whisk the eggs, water, oregano, salt, black pepper, and butter and combine well.
4. Fold in coconut flour and baking soda.
5. Mix in the parmesan and feta cheese, olives, spinach, and red pepper until combined.
6. Spoon the mixture into the cups and bake for 12-15 minutes until golden and a skewer comes out clean. Serve and enjoy!

Nutrition per serving (2 mini muffins)

Calories: 190

- Total Fat 15.3g
- Saturated Fat 8.1g
- Cholesterol 138mg
- Sodium 324mg
- Total Carbohydrate 6.5g
- Dietary Fiber 3.4g
- Total Sugars 1g
- Protein 7.6g

Tomato Pesto Tart with Cauliflower Crust

Your new go-to dinner party starter, your midweek dinner, packed lunch, and new favorite tart. Enjoy this guilt-free, gluten-free and grain-free treat however you choose!

Serves: 6

Ingredients

- 12 oz cauliflower florets
- 1 cup grated mozzarella cheese
- 1 large egg beaten
- 1 tsp oregano
- ¾ tsp minced fresh garlic
- ¼ tsp turmeric
- ¼ tsp salt
- ⅛ tsp cayenne pepper
- ¼ cup pesto
- ½ cup crumbled goat cheese
- 2 ripe thinly sliced tomatoes
- ¼ tsp crushed red pepper flakes or more to taste optional
- 4 Tbsp fresh basil (chopped)

Method

1. Preheat the oven to 425F and prepare a baking sheet.
2. Blend your cauliflower florets in a food processor until you achieve a grain-like consistency.
3. Cook the cauliflower on high in the microwave for 7 minutes.
4. Remove from the microwave and stir, carefully letting the steam escape and leave it to cool slightly.
5. Mix together the cauliflower, mozzarella, egg, oregano, garlic, turmeric, salt, and cayenne pepper. Stir until well combined.
6. On your baking sheet, press out the mixture to form a 10-inch circle of even thickness, making sure to keep the center as thin as the edges. This will be your cauliflower base! Create a small crust around the edge with your fingers.
7. Bake for 20 minutes.
    i. Remove from the oven and leave to cool. Evenly spread the pesto before covering in the goat's cheese, tomatoes, and red pepper flakes.
    ii. Place the tart under a hot grill for 3-4 minutes until hot and bubbly.
    iii. Remove and sprinkle with fresh basil and enjoy warm or cold!

Nutrition per serving

Calories: 181

- Total Fat 13g
- Saturated Fat 6g
- Cholesterol 55mg
- Sodium 412mg
- Total Carbohydrate 6g
- Dietary Fiber 1g
- Total Sugars 2g
- Protein 10g

Dark Chocolate and Sea Salt Cookies

Name one thing more comforting and delicious than a chocolate chip cookie... a keto chocolate chip cookie. This five-step recipe is as simple and tasty as it sounds, perfect for making for drop-in guests, late night cravings or family 'emergencies'.

Serves: 10

Ingredients

- 1 cup finely ground almond flour
- 2-4 Tbsp sugar-free chocolate chips
- 2 Tbsp powdered erythritol
- 1/8 tsp baking soda
- 2 Tbsp coconut oil
- 1 tsp pure vanilla extract
- 3 tsp milk
- 1/2 tsp sea salt flakes

Method

1. Preheat oven to 325F and prepare a baking sheet.
2. Stir the flour, chocolate, and sugar until well combined.
3. Add the wet ingredients to form a thick dough.

4. Shape into cookies and sprinkle with sea salt flakes before placing on your baking sheet, and bake for 10 minutes and golden brown.

5. Leave to cool and firm up as much as you can before eating, or enjoy soft and warm with a spoon if you can't wait (we're not judging)!

Nutrition per serving

Calories: 115

- Total Fat 10.2g
- Saturated Fat 3.5g
- Cholesterol 2mg
- Sodium 74mg
- Total Carbohydrate 5.7g
- Dietary Fiber 2.2g
- Total Sugars 0.5g
- Protein 2.9g

Garlic and Cheese Crackers

When it gets to 3 pm and you are desperate for a snack, you need a Tupperware box of these cheesy garlic crackers! Add to a fruit platter, cheese board or nibble throughout the day for a quick and easy treat.

Serves: 12

Ingredients

- 3 Tbsp coconut flour
- ¼ tsp salt
- ½ tsp garlic powder
- ½ tsp dried oregano
- ¼ tsp baking powder
- 2 Tbsp butter (soft)
- ½ cup mozzarella cheese (grated)
- ¼ cup water

Method

1. Preheat the oven to 400F and prepare a baking sheet.
2. Mix the coconut flour, salt, garlic, oregano, and baking powder together in a large bowl until well combined.
3. Add the butter and blend well then mix in the cheese

and water until a dough forms.

4. Lay the dough out between two sheets of parchment paper and roll out to about ¼ inch thick.

5. Cut into squares and poke with a fork.

6. Bake for 13 - 16 minutes until golden and firm.

Nutrition per serving

Calories: 36

- Total Fat 2.5g
- Saturated Fat 1.6g
- Cholesterol 6mg
- Sodium 71mg
- Total Carbohydrate 2.1g
- Dietary Fiber 1.5g
- Total Sugars 0g
- Protein 0.9g

Rosemary and Sea Salt Focaccia

All the soft and chewy goodness of a classic Italian Focaccia with as much olive oil, rosemary and sea salt as you can eat!

Serves: 9

Ingredients

- 2 tsp active dry yeast
- 2 tsp honey (this is to feed the yeast and no sugar will remain post bake)
- 80 ml water
- 144g almond flour
- 28g psyllium husk (finely ground)
- 1 Tbsp ground flax seeds
- 1 ½ tsp baking powder
- ½ tsp sea salt
- 1 egg at room temperature
- 2 egg whites at room temperature
- 13g extra virgin olive oil
- 2 tsp apple cider vinegar

For the topping

- rosemary springs
- extra virgin olive oil
- flakey sea salt

Method

1. Mix yeast and maple syrup to a large bowl.
2. Heat up the water to 110F and pour over the yeast mixture, cover bowl with a kitchen towel and allow to rest for 7 minutes. The mixture should start to bubble up!
3. To a medium bowl, add almond flour, psyllium husk, flax seeds, baking powder, and salt and mix until thoroughly mixed.
4. With an electric whisk, blend the egg, egg whites, olive oil, and vinegar to the proofed yeast. Then, adding a small amount at a time, mix in the flour until well incorporated and a dough is formed.
5. Grease a baking sheet with olive oil and spread the dough to cover the sheet to an even thickness. The dough will be sticky, so wet your fingers before touching it! Make indentations in the dough and fill with rosemary springs and follow with a generous drizzle of olive oil and a sprinkle of sea salt. Cover with cling film and place in a warm, dark space for 40-50 minutes until lighter in texture and slightly raised. Preheat your oven to 350F while the dough is

proofing.

6.

7. Transfer the baking sheet gently into the oven and bake for 25-30 minutes. Cover with foil halfway through if it's starting to color too quickly.

8. After removing from the oven, leave to cool for 30 minutes for the best texture and enjoy!

Nutrition per serving (before toppings have been added)

Calories: 259

- Total Fat 6.7g
- Saturated Fat 0.6g
- Cholesterol 0mg
- Sodium 151mg
- Total Carbohydrate 7.3g
- Dietary Fiber 3.9g
- Total Sugars 1.3g
- Protein 3.9g

Mojito Cupcakes

Who says cocktails need to be saved for Friday? Enjoy these delicate and flavorsome mojito cupcakes day or night to instantly inject some fun to your week.

Serves: 10

Ingredients

Sponge

- 1 cup almond flour
- 2 Tbsp coconut flour
- 1 tsp baking powder
- ½ tsp sea salt
- 1 cup heavy whipping cream
- 2 whole eggs
- 4 egg yolks
- ¼ cup powdered stevia
- ½ tsp liquid stevia
- ½ tsp vanilla bean paste
- zest of 1 lime

Frosting

- ½ cup butter (softened)
- 2 Tbsp coconut oil

- 2 Tbsp powdered stevia
- zest of 1 lime
- 2 tsp rum

Garnish

- fresh mint leaves and lime slices

Method

1. Preheat the oven to 350F and prepare a muffin pan with 10 liners.
2. Mix the almond flour, coconut flour, baking powder, and salt in a bowl.
3. Use an electric mixer to whip the cream to soft peaks and slowly add in the eggs and yolks, one at a time. When well combined, mix in the powdered stevia, liquid stevia, vanilla, and lime zest.
4. Fold the flour mixture into the sweetened cream.
5. Fill each liner with the cupcake batter and bake for 20 minutes, once baked, remove to cool completely before frosting.

Frosting

1. Use an electric mixer to whisk the butter, sugar and coconut oil until light and fluffy before adding the rum and lime zest.
2. When the cupcakes are cool, add your frosting with a

knife or pipe it on for a more curated finish. Decorate with mint leaves and lime slices for extra finesse!

Nutrition per serving

Calories: 259

- Total Fat 24.5g
- Saturated Fat 12.4g
- Cholesterol 157mg
- Sodium 184mg
- Total Carbohydrate 5.2g
- Dietary Fiber 2g
- Total Sugars 0.5g
- Protein 5.2g

Rosemary Cheddar Cornbread

Using a skillet creates a moreish crust on this light and fluffy cornbread. The aromatic rosemary and tangy cheddar is a match made in heaven for breakfast, lunch, and dinner. On the unlikely chance that you have leftovers, this versatile bread will stay fresh for up to 4 days in a Tupperware container.

Serves: 16

Ingredients

- ½ cup almond flour
- ¼ cup coconut flour
- 1 tsp salt
- ½ tsp baking soda
- 3 large eggs
- ½ cup heavy cream
- ¼ cup butter (melted)
- 2 Tbsp rosemary (chopped)
- ½ cup cheddar cheese (shredded)

Method

1. Preheat the oven to 325F and prepare a cast iron skillet.

2. Simply mix together all of the ingredients in a medium bowl until well combined.

3. Pour the batter into the skillet and bake for 25-30 minutes!

Nutrition per serving

Calories: 96

- **Total Fat** 8.3g
- Saturated Fat 4g
- **Cholesterol** 51mg
- **Sodium** 244mg
- **Total Carbohydrate** 2.5g
- Dietary Fiber 1.3g
- Total Sugars 0.1g
- **Protein** 3.2g

Jalapeno Popper Pittas

Jalapeno popper pittas are as fun to make as they're to eat! The mild and tangy heat, blended into cooling cream cheese melts together with these fresh and crispy pitta breads.

Serves: 5

Ingredients

Pittas

- 2 eggs
- 2 tsp baking powder
- ½ tsp sea salt
- 2 cups of finely shredded mozzarella cheese
- 1.5 cups almond flour

Filling

- 200g cream cheese
- 1 fresh jalapeno (seeds removed)

Method

1. Preheat the oven to 400F and prepare a baking sheet.

2. In a large bowl, beat the eggs and add the salt and baking powder. Then mix in cheese and almond flour.

3. Put some oil on your hands and separate the dough into 5 equal balls. Flatten each ball and spread them out on a piece of parchment paper and place another piece of parchment paper on top. Use a rolling pin to flatten each dough until they are about 5-6 inches in diameter.

4. Transfer the dough and bottom piece of parchment to a sheet tray and bake for 13-15 minutes. Remove and set aside to cool.

5. Mix the cream cheese and jalapenos together in a bowl and spread on top of the pitta bread!

Nutrition per serving

Calories: 250

- Total Fat 21.7g
- Saturated Fat 10.8g
- Cholesterol 115mg
- Sodium 410mg
- Total Carbohydrate 4.5g
- Dietary Fiber 1g
- Total Sugars 0.3g
- Protein 10.3g

Chocolate Donuts

Light and rich chocolate donuts, dipped in a sweet and decadent glaze - perfection.

Serves: 8

Ingredients

Donuts

- ⅓ cup coconut flour
- ⅓ cup stevia
- 3 Tbsp cocoa powder
- 1 tsp baking powder
- ¼ tsp salt
- 4 large eggs
- ¼ cup butter (melted)
- ½ tsp vanilla extract
- 6 Tbsp brewed coffee

Glaze

- ¼ cup powdered stevia
- 1 Tbsp cocoa powder
- 1 Tbsp heavy cream
- ¼ tsp vanilla extract
- 1 ½ Tbsp water

Method

1. Preheat the oven to 325F and grease a donut pan.

2. In a medium-sized bowl, whisk together the coconut flour, stevia, cocoa powder, baking powder, and salt. Then mix in the eggs, melted butter, vanilla extract, and cold coffee until well combined.

3. Fill the donut pan with the batter and bake 16-20 minutes. Remove and let cool completely.

4. Mix together the powdered stevia and cocoa powder. Add the heavy cream and vanilla and whisk until combined.

5. Add enough water until the glaze thins out and is wet enough to dip the donuts into the glaze, once dipped, leave to set for 30 minutes.

Nutrition per serving

Calories: 121

- Total Fat 9.8g
- Saturated Fat 5.4g
- Cholesterol 111mg
- Sodium 152mg
- Total Carbohydrate 5.4g
- Dietary Fiber 2.8g
- Total Sugars 0.3g
- Protein 4.4g

Rye Bread

This flavorsome loaf makes unbelievable sandwiches or perfect toast for days and days. Please note that this recipe is designed for a small loaf pan, so double your portion size and the nutritional information if you're feeling hungry!

Serves: 8

Ingredients

- 1 cup almond flour
- ¾ cup brown flaxmeal
- ½ tsp sea salt
- ½ tsp baking soda
- ¾ tsp cream of tartar
- 3 large eggs
- 2 Tbsp olive oil
- ¼ cup water
- 2 Tbsp caraway seeds

Method

1. Preheat the oven to 350F and prepare a loaf pan.
2. In a large bowl combine almond flour, flax, salt, baking soda, and cream of tartar.

3. In a small bowl combine eggs, oil, and water.
4. Stir the wet ingredients into the dry, then mix in caraway seeds.
5. Allow batter to sit for 2 minutes to thicken. Then transfer the batter into the loaf pan.
6. Bake for 35-45 minutes and cool for 1 hour.

Nutrition per serving

Calories: 149

- Total Fat 11.9g
- Saturated Fat 1.2g
- Cholesterol 70mg
- Sodium 229mg
- Total Carbohydrate 6.6g
- Dietary Fiber 4.8g
- Total Sugars 0.2g
- Protein 6.2g

Cauliflower Breadsticks

Transform your movie night with these cauliflower breadsticks and dip them into salsa, guac or any dip of your choice. Make them as cheesy and garlicky as you please and enjoy your new favorite finger food!

Serves: 2

Ingredients

- 2 cups cauliflower (riced)
- 1 Tbsp butter
- 3 tsp garlic (minced)
- ¼ tsp red pepper flakes
- ½ tsp Italian herbs
- ¼ tsp sea salt
- 1 cup mozzarella (shredded)
- 1 egg
- ¼ cup grated parmesan (dried)

Method

1. Preheat the oven to 350F and prepare a baking sheet.
2. Microwave your cauliflower for 3 minutes and melt butter in a small skillet over low heat adding garlic and

red pepper flakes and mixing for 3 minutes, being careful not to let it brown.

3. Add the seasoned butter to the bowl of cooked cauliflower and mix in herbs and salt to the bowl.
4. Chill for 10 minutes so the egg doesn't cook, then add the egg and mozzarella to your mixture.
5. Press the cauliflower mix into your baking sheet until evenly distributed.
6. Bake for 30 minutes and take out of the oven to sprinkle with parmesan (and extra mozzarella if you're as cheese obsessed as we are) then return to the oven for an additional 8 minutes. Leave to cool and slice into strips or 'breadsticks'!

Nutrition per serving

Calories: 173

- Total Fat 13.5g
- Saturated Fat 7.7g
- Cholesterol 114mg
- Sodium 547mg
- Total Carbohydrate 2.8g
- Dietary Fiber 0.2g
- Total Sugars 0.4g
- Protein 11.2g

Zucchini Pizza

Fear not, a keto diet certainly doesn't mean pizza needs to be taken off your food plan - what kind of a life would that be?

Serves: 6

Ingredients

- 3 cups zucchini (grated)
- ⅔ cup almond flour
- 2 Tbsp coconut flour
- 3 Tbsp nutritional yeast
- 1 Tbsp Italian seasoning
- ½ tsp salt
- 2 large eggs (beaten)

Add any keto toppings of your choice, we love pesto chicken, garlicky seafood or just a good ol' margarita!

Method

1. Preheat the oven to 400F and prepare a baking sheet.
2. Add the grated zucchini to the center of a clean dish towel and squeeze out all of the liquid. Once no more liquid appears, transfer it to a medium-sized bowl.

3. Then mix in the flours, nutritional yeast, and seasoning and until thoroughly combined.
4. Finally, add the eggs and stir to form a sticky dough. Transfer the dough to the baking sheet and spread the mixture out using your hands to form a thin and even pizza base. If it's too sticky you can use water or oil on your fingertips!
5. Bake for 20 minutes, then flip your base around and bake for a further 10. Remove from the oven and top with your desired toppings, then bake for a final 10 minutes until the toppings are cooked. To get a crispy crust, leave to cool and firm for 10 minutes once removed from the oven and then slice and serve!

Nutrition per serving

Calories: 153

- Total Fat 9.1g
- Saturated Fat 1.5g
- Cholesterol 64mg
- Sodium 231mg
- Total Carbohydrate 10.6g
- Dietary Fiber 5.2g
- Total Sugars 1.4g
- Protein 8.4g

Chocolate and Peanut Butter Protein Balls

These protein balls or 'fat bombs' are chewy, chocolaty and oh so peanutty.

Serves: 45

Ingredients

- 2 cups peanut butter (smooth works best)
- 3 cups almond flour
- ⅓ cup yacon syrup
- 1 ½ cups 100% chocolate (chopped)

Method

1. Prepare a baking sheet.
2. Mix the peanut butter, coconut flour, and syrup together until combined. If the batter is too dry you can add a few teaspoons of water.
3. Turn the batter into small balls and place on the tray and freeze for 10 minutes.
4. Melt the chocolate pieces in a Bain-marie. Remove the protein balls from the freezer and drizzle with the

melted chocolate.

5. When the chocolate is dried up, enjoy!

Nutrition per serving

Calories: 143

- Total Fat 12.4g
- Saturated Fat 3.6g
- Cholesterol 0mg
- Sodium 57mg
- Total Carbohydrate 6.6g
- Dietary Fiber 2.5g
- Total Sugars 1.9g
- Protein 5.3g

Cloud Bread

There's a reason why it's called cloud bread, this keto favorite is lighter than air and melts in the mouth!

Serves: 8

Ingredients

- 3 large eggs (room temperature)
- ¼ tsp cream of tartar
- pinch of sea salt
- ½ cup cream cheese (softened)

Method

1. Preheat the oven to 300F and prepare a baking sheet.
2. Separate egg whites from yolks into two glass bowls.
3. To the egg whites, add cream of tartar and salt, then using an electric mixer, beat until stiff peaks form. Add cream cheese to egg yolks and mix until well combined. Gently fold the yolk into the whites.
4. Divide mixture into 8 circles on your baking sheet and bake for 25 to 30 minutes.

5. Sprinkle with any ingredients you like or enjoy plain!

Nutrition per serving

Calories: 78

- Total Fat 6.9g
- Saturated Fat 3.8g
- Cholesterol 86mg
- Sodium 100mg
- Total Carbohydrate 0.6g
- Dietary Fiber 0g
- Total Sugars 0.2g
- Protein 3.5g

Lavender Shortbread

These delicate lavender cookies taste like they were created for an English country garden and afternoon tea with a cuppa! For extra presentation points, add a lavender colored glaze and some lavender pieces or springs, picture perfect and deliciously fragrant.

Serves: 20

Ingredients

- 2 tsp dried lavender
- ⅓ cup coconut flour
- ⅔ cup almond flour
- ¼ cup granulated erythritol
- 8 drops liquid Stevia
- ½ cup butter (softened)
- 1 tsp vanilla extract
- ¼ tsp baking powder
- ¼ tsp xanthan gum

Method

1. Preheat the oven to 355F and prepare a baking sheet.

2. Using a pestle and mortar, finely grind the lavender until it is almost a powder.
3. Mix together your dry ingredients then add softened butter, vanilla extract, and stevia and combine until you form a dough.
4. Wrap your dough up in Clingfilm and refrigerate for 10 minutes to firm up.
5. Use a cookie cutter to cut out as many shapes and pieces of shortbread as you can and place them on your baking sheet.
6. Bake for 6 minutes or until firm, leave the cookies to cool completely and enjoy!

Nutrition per serving

Calories: 72

- Total Fat 6.6g
- Saturated Fat 3.2g
- Cholesterol 12mg
- Sodium 37mg
- Total Carbohydrate 5.3g
- Dietary Fiber 1.3g
- Total Sugars 3g
- Protein 1.1g

Pepperoni Pizza Quiche

Two of our favorite foods, pizza and quiche. A modern twist on a picnic classic and as customizable as you like!

Serves: 6

Ingredients

- 2 tsp olive oil
- 2 ½ cups mushrooms (sliced)
- 1 cup of peppers (sliced)
- 1 cup olives (sliced)
- 1 cup mozzarella cheese (shredded)
- 1 cup pizza cheese (shredded)
- 2 tsp dried Italian herb
- 4 eggs (beaten)
- ½ cup heavy cream
- ¼ tsp garlic powder
- ¾ cup sliced pepperoni

Method

1. Preheat oven to 400F and prepare a pie dish.

2. Use an oiled pan to fry the mushrooms and peppers on medium heat until lightly browned.
3. Combine the cheese and herbs in a bowl and place in a pie dish.
4. Beat together the eggs then mix in the heavy cream, and eventually the cheese in the pie dish.
5. Make a layer of mushrooms, peppers, and olives on top of the cheesy egg mix.
6. Cover with pepperoni and add more herbs.
7. Bake the quiche 30-35 minutes, or until the eggs are completely set and the pepperoni is starting to brown.
8. Let the quiche cool 3-5 minutes and enjoy!

Nutrition per serving

Calories: 266

- Total Fat 20.9g
- Saturated Fat 9.2g
- Cholesterol 154mg
- Sodium 583mg
- Total Carbohydrate g
- Dietary Fiber 8.1g
- Total Sugars 0.8g
- Protein 14.5g

Squid Ink Rolls

These jet black rolls make striking sandwiches which your guests will not believe you made from scratch! We love dusting ours with some coconut flour for a beautiful contrast but you can also add sesame seeds before baking for a similar effect.

Serves: 6

Ingredients

- 5 Tbsp ground psyllium husk powder
- 1¼ cups almond flour
- 2 tsp baking powder
- 1 tsp sea salt
- 2 tsp cider vinegar
- 3 egg whites
- 1 cup water
- 2 Tbsp squid ink

Method

1. Preheat the oven to 350F and prepare a baking sheet.
2. Mix the dry ingredients in a large bowl and bring the water to a boil.

3. Mix together the vinegar and egg whites with the dry ingredients. Add boiling water and squid ink while beating with a hand mixer until combined and a dough is formed.
4. Season your hands with a little olive oil and shape the dough into 6 separate rolls. Carefully place on your sheet.
5. Bake for 1 hour!

Nutrition per serving

Calories: 389

- Total Fat 24.4g
- Saturated Fat 1.8g
- Cholesterol 0mg
- Sodium 420mg
- Total Carbohydrate 40.1g
- Dietary Fiber 29g
- Total Sugars 0.1g
- Protein 12.8g

Cardamom, Rose and Pistachio Scones

Floral and aromatic, every mouthful of these buttery scones is a journey of flavor. Perfectly delectable alone or even more luxe with cream or butter or jam or all 3!

Serves: 12

Ingredients

- 1 ½ cups almond flour
- 1 Tbsp baking powder
- ½ tsp ground cardamom
- 1 Tbsp dried rose petals
- ¼ cup chopped pistachios
- 4 Tbsp unsalted butter (softened)
- 2 large eggs
- ⅓ cup sour cream
- 1 tsp rose water
- 2 Tbsp coconut milk

Method

1. Preheat the oven to 390F and prepare a muffin tray.
2. In a large bowl mix together the dry ingredients.
3. Add softened butter, eggs, sour cream, and rose water

and stir to combine.

4. Add the wet ingredients to the dry and mix thoroughly, ensuring everything is evenly combined. Use your hands and have fun!
5. Scoop heaped tablespoons of the batter into the muffin tins and wash the tops with milk.
6. Bake for 10 minutes until golden brown.

Nutrition per serving

Calories: 157

- Total Fat 13.9g
- Saturated Fat 4.6g
- Cholesterol 44mg
- Sodium 55mg
- Total Carbohydrate 4.4g
- Dietary Fiber 1.7g
- Total Sugars 0.2g
- Protein 4.6g

Pumpkin Pie

Autumn in a mouthful. The kind of pie you make with intentions of eating for dessert and end up eating for breakfast, lunch, and dinner - no regrets.

Serves: 12

Ingredients

Pie crust

- 2 ½ cup blanched almond flour
- ⅓ cup erythritol
- ¼ tsp sea salt
- ¼ cup ghee (measured solid, then melted)
- 1 large egg

Pumpkin filling

- 1 15-oz can pumpkin puree
- ½ cup heavy cream
- 2 large eggs
- 1 tsp blackstrap molasses
- ⅔ cup powdered erythritol
- 2 tsp pumpkin pie spice

- ¼ tsp sea salt
- 1 tsp vanilla extract

Method

1. Preheat the oven to 350F and prepare a pie pan.
2. In a large bowl, mix together the almond flour, erythritol and sea salt.
3. Stir in the melted ghee, vanilla, and egg, until well combined and a dough is formed.
4. Press the dough into the bottom of the prepared pan, fluting the sides if preferred. Poke holes in the surface using a fork.
5. Bake for 10 minutes, until lightly golden and leave to cool whilst preparing your filling. Lower the oven to 325F.
6. Beat together the remaining ingredients until smooth and fill the cooled crust. Gently tap on the counter to release air bubbles.
7. Bake for 45 minutes until the pie is almost set but still slightly soft.
8. Cool completely then refrigerate. Serve with a sprinkle of cinnamon and whipped cream.

Nutrition per serving

Calories: 237

- Total Fat 18.6g
- Saturated Fat 5.1g
- Cholesterol 64mg
- Sodium 91mg
- Total Carbohydrate 26.9g
- Dietary Fiber 3.7g
- Total Sugars 3.4g
- Protein 7.2g

Salted Caramel Apple Tart

A classic apple tart, just like grandma used to make, but with a sweet and salted caramel twist!

Serves: 8

Ingredients

Base

- 6 Tbsp butter (melted)
- 2 cups almond flour
- ⅓ cup erythritol sweetener
- 1 tsp nutmeg

Filling

- ½ cup salted caramel
- 3 cups thinly sliced Granny Smith apples (peeled and cored)
- 2 tsp lemon juice
- ¼ cup butter
- ½ tsp ground cinnamon
- ¼ cup erythritol sweetener
- 2 tsp lemon zest

Method

1. Preheat the oven to 375F and prepare a pie dish.
2. Combine butter, almond flour, sweetener, and nutmeg in a medium-sized bowl until combined.
3. Press the dough firmly into the dish and up to the edges to create a crust. Pre-bake the crust for 5 minutes.
4. Combine the sliced apples, lemon zest and lemon juice in a medium bowl and lay them evenly across the bottom of the crust. Press the apples down lightly when done.
5. Combine the butter, cinnamon, and sweetener in a small bowl and microwave for 1 minute, cover with apples and then drizzle with salted caramel sauce.
6. Bake the tart for 30 minutes and reduce the heat to 350F to bake the tart for another 20 minutes, remove from the oven and enjoy!

Nutrition per serving

Calories: 393

- Total Fat 28g
- Saturated Fat 10.2g
- Cholesterol 38mg
- Sodium 145mg

- Total Carbohydrate 31.5g
- Dietary Fiber 5.4g
- Total Sugars 8.9g
- Protein 6.7g

Cheese and Pesto Pinwheels

Cheesy pesto pinwheels with none of the mess. These muffin-tart crossbreeds are full of flavor, quick to make and far too easy to eat.

Serves: 8

Ingredients

Dough

- ¾ cup almond flour
- ½ tsp baking powder
- 1 ½ cups mozzarella cheese (shredded)
- ⅛ cup cream cheese
- 1 large egg beaten

Filling

- ⅓ cup pesto
- 1 cup cheddar cheese (shredded)
- ¼ cup red pepper (roasted)
- ¼ cup red onion (sliced)

Method

1. Preheat the oven to 375F and prepare a muffin tray.
2. Mix almond flour and baking powder in a bowl.
3. Melt the mozzarella and cream cheese together in a bain-marie until smooth.
4. Add the egg into the cheese mix and stir in the almond flour. Knead to create a dough.
5. Roll the dough out between 2 sheets of parchment paper to a large, even rectangle.
6. Cover the top with pesto, leaving a border of about 1 inch along the outside. Add cheese, red pepper, and red onion.
7. Use the parchment to roll up the dough into a log. Cut the log into 8 equal pieces.
8. Place a roll into each muffin wells and bake until golden, about 25 to 30 minutes. Cool slightly before serving and serve with a dollop of Greek yogurt for a Sunday morning treat!

Nutrition per serving

Calories: 196

- Total Fat 16.2g
- Saturated Fat 5.6g

- Cholesterol 24mg
- Sodium 212mg
- Total Carbohydrate 4.2g
- Dietary Fiber 1.5g
- Total Sugars 1.2g
- Protein 8.6g

Gingerbread Men

Reminisce about simpler times with these traditional gingerbread men. Ice on outfits, stick on sweets, dust with powdered sugar or just munch away. Legs or head first?

Serves: 18

Ingredients

- ½ butter (melted)
- ¾ erythritol
- 1 whole egg + 1 egg yolk
- 2 ½ Tbs coconut flour
- ⅞ almond flour
- 1 Tbs baking powder
- ½ tsp xanthan gum
- ½ Tbs ground ginger
- ½ Tbs mixed spice

Method

1. Preheat the oven to 335F and prepare a baking sheet.
2. Mix together the butter, erythritol and 1 whole egg until well combined.

3. In a separate bowl, mix together your dry ingredients and mix thoroughly. Stir in the egg yolk.
4. Combine the butter mix and dry ingredients and wrap up in cellophane to firm up and refrigerate for 1 hour.
5. Roll to 5mm thickness and use a cookie cutter to make as many shapes as you can. Bake for 10 - 12 minutes. Enjoy warm and crumbly out of the oven or allow to cool for a firmer cookie.

Nutrition per serving

Calories: 37

- Total Fat 2.9g
- Saturated Fat 1.3g
- Cholesterol 24mg
- Sodium 18mg
- Total Carbohydrate 1.9g
- Dietary Fiber 0.7g
- Total Sugars 0.3g
- Protein 1.3g

Sundried Tomato Bread

We love this fragrant sundried tomato bread toasted with butter or dipped in pumpkin soup.

Serves: 10

Ingredients

- 255g ground almonds
- 1 Tbsp Oregano
- ½ tsp erythritol
- ¼ tsp sea salt
- ½ tsp baking soda
- ¼ cup flax seeds
- 2 sprigs of thyme
- ½ tsp cracked black pepper
- ¼ cup almond milk
- 1 tsp apple cider vinegar
- 1 Tbsp olive oil
- 1 Tbsp yogurt
- 2 large eggs
- 25g sundried tomatoes

Method

1. Preheat the oven to 330F and line a loaf tin.
2. Mix the dry ingredients together.
3. Add the wet ingredients and form a smooth batter, then mix in the tomatoes.
4. Fill the loaf tin and bake for 35 minutes.

Nutrition per serving

Calories: 217

- Total Fat 18g
- Saturated Fat 3g
- Cholesterol 37mg
- Sodium 201mg
- Total Carbohydrate 9.1g
- Dietary Fiber 4.8g
- Total Sugars 2.7g
- Protein 7.9g

Rainbow Cinnamon Rolls

The Swedish specialty with a colorful makeover. These cinnamon rolls look like they have taken much longer than they have and give you instant brownie points with the kids!

Serves: 12

Ingredients

- 1 ½ cup mozzarella (shredded)
- ¾ cup almond flour
- 2 Tbsp cream cheese
- 1 egg
- ½ tsp baking powder
- 2 Tbsp rainbow sprinkles (sugar-free)

Filling

- 2 Tbsp water
- 2 Tbsp granulated stevia
- 2 tsp cinnamon

Topping

- 2 Tbsp cream cheese
- 1 Tbsp yogurt

- 2 drops vanilla stevia
- 2 Tbsp rainbow sprinkles (sugar-free)

Method

1. Preheat the oven to 360F and prepare a baking dish.
2. Melt the mozzarella and cream cheese in the microwave for 1 ½ minutes, stirring halfway through and stir in the egg.
3. Now add the almond flour and baking powder and knead to make a dough.
4. Divide the dough into 6 even balls and form long rolls. Then flatten out with your hands to make the dough as thin as possible.
5. To make your cinnamon filling, boil water, sweetener and cinnamon. Spread over the flattened dough rolls.
6. Roll each into a bun and cut sideways in half to make 12 rolls, place on the baking dish and bake for 20 minutes.
7. While the rolls are in the oven, prepare the frosting by combining cream cheese, yogurt, and stevia.
8. Drizzle over the warm rolls, sprinkle with the final serving of rainbow sprinkles and serve!

Nutrition per serving

Calories: 86

- Total Fat 5.5g
- Saturated Fat 1.5g
- Cholesterol 19mg
- Sodium 40mg
- Total Carbohydrate 6.9g
- Dietary Fiber 1g
- Total Sugars 4.8g
- Protein 3.3g

Gruyère, Onion and Thyme Tear & Share

These soft and fluffy rolls are filled with aromatic thyme, salty gruyère, and sweet red onions. Once it's baked you can serve in the middle of the table or add to a buffet and let everybody tear and share!

Serves: 16

Ingredients

- 2 ½ cups mozzarella (grated)
- 3 eggs (beaten)
- 1 ½ cups almond flour
- 1 Tbsp baking powder
- ¼ cup cream cheese
- ½ cup parmesan (grated)
- 2 red onions (thinly sliced)
- 140g gruyère (grated)
- 1 Tbsp thyme leaves

Method

1. Preheat the oven to 350F and prepare a bundt pan.
2. Combine the almond flour with the baking powder in one bowl then melt the mozzarella and cream cheese

for 1 minute in the microwave in another.

3. Combine these two mixes and add eggs until combined then knead until it's all come together from the sides of the bowl. It should be nice and sticky at this stage so sprinkle with a little parmesan to make it easier to handle.
4. Roll out 30 even sized balls of dough.
5. On a large plate add the remaining parmesan and thyme and roll each ball of dough onto the plate until covered.
6. Cover the pan with 15 balls then cover with half the gruyere and red onion, then repeat on top.
7. Bake for 25 minutes or until golden, tear your pieces away and enjoy!

Nutrition per serving

Calories: 158

- Total Fat 11.7g
- Saturated Fat 4.2g
- Cholesterol 50mg
- Sodium 127mg
- Total Carbohydrate 4.6g
- Dietary Fiber 1.5g
- Total Sugars 0.7g
- Protein 9.1g

Coffee Cake

Upgrade your afternoon coffee for this sweet and creamy sponge cake and eradicate the 3 pm slump.

Serves: 16

Ingredients

Cake

- 3 cups almond flour
- ¾ cup monk fruit sweetener
- ½ cup unsweetened almond milk
- 3 large eggs
- ½ cup butter (melted)
- 1 Tbsp instant coffee dissolved in 1 Tbsp hot water

Frosting

- 3 Tbsp cream cheese (softened)
- 1 Tbsp heavy whipping cream
- 2 Tbsp monk fruit sweetener
- 1 Tbsp instant coffee dissolved in 1 Tbsp hot water

Method

1. Preheat the oven to 350F and prepare a baking pan.
2. In a large bowl mix all of the cake ingredients until well combined.
3. Fill the pan with your cake mix and bake in the oven for 35 minutes.
4. Mix the cream cheese, whipping cream and sweetener then slowly add in the coffee (making sure it's cooled completely).
5. Remove the cake from the oven and allow to cool before piping on the frosting. Garnish with coffee beans if you have them or sugar-free cocoa powder.

Nutrition per serving

Calories: 201

- Total Fat 17.8g
- Saturated Fat 5.3g
- Cholesterol 53mg
- Sodium 73mg
- Total Carbohydrate 15.7g
- Dietary Fiber 2.3g
- Total Sugars 0.1g
- Protein 5.9g

Cheese, Garlic and Red Pesto Twists

These easy to make and easier to eat cheesy twists make ideal breakfasts, lunches or sides to a dinner.

Serves: 10

Ingredients

- ½ cup almond flour
- 4 Tbsp coconut flour
- ½ tsp salt
- 1 tsp baking powder
- 1½ cups mozzarella (shredded)
- ⅓ cup butter
- 1 egg
- ¼ red pesto
- 1 egg (for brushing the top)
- 1 tsp red pepper flakes
- 1 tsp garlic granules

Method

1. Preheat the oven to 350F and prepare a baking tray.

2. Mix together all dry ingredients.
3. Melt the butter and the cheese together on low heat then add the eggs and combine until smooth.
4. Combine the mixes until a firm dough is formed.
5. Using a piece of parchment paper on each side of the dough, use a rolling pin to roll out into a rectangle shape.
6. Take the top piece of paper away and spread with pesto before cutting into strips and twist the strips and carefully place on the baking sheet.
7. Brush the twists with whisked egg then sprinkle the pepper flakes, garlic granules, and any other seasoning.
8. Bake for 15–20 minutes until they're golden brown and leave to cool and crisp up!

Nutrition per serving

Calories: 162

- Total Fat 13.1g
- Saturated Fat 6.2g
- Cholesterol 57mg
- Sodium 273mg
- Total Carbohydrate 4.4g
- Dietary Fiber 1.9g
- Total Sugars 0.1g
- Protein 7.3g

Poppy Seed Bagels

Because nobody should miss out on the humble and satisfying bagel, whatever their diet. These poppy seed, keto versions are full of New York nostalgia and flavor.

Serves: 6

Ingredients

- 1 ½ cup mozzarella (shredded)
- 2 Tbsp cream cheese (full fat)
- ¼ cup coconut flour
- 1 egg
- 1 tsp baking powder
- ¼ tsp sea salt
- 1 Tbsp almond milk
- 2 Tbsp poppy seeds

Method

1. Preheat the oven to 425F and prepare a baking sheet.
2. Mix the mozzarella, cream cheese, and coconut flour into a microwaveable bowl and heat for 1 minute. Stir then heat for a further 30 seconds.

3. Mix together the egg, baking powder, and salt.

4. Divide the dough into 6 equal portions and roll into cylinder shapes. Then fold the cylinder shapes into a circle and squeeze the two ends together to form a bagel.

5. Place on the baking tray and brush with milk, then sprinkle with poppy seeds. Bake for 15 minutes, or until golden brown.

Nutrition per serving

Calories: 84

- Total Fat 5.6g
- Saturated Fat 2.7g
- Cholesterol 35mg
- Sodium 142mg
- Total Carbohydrate 5g
- Dietary Fiber 2.4g
- Total Sugars 0.6g
- Protein 4.4g

Chocolate Pistachio Shortbread

Buttery shortbread with aromatic pistachios and smothered in chocolate... yes please!

Serves: 16

Ingredients

Shortbread

- 6 Tbsp butter (melted)
- 2 cups superfine almond flour
- ½ cup powdered erythritol sweetener
- ½ cup chopped pistachios
- 1 tsp vanilla extract

Garnish

- ¾ cup sugar-free dark chocolate

Method

1. Preheat the oven to 350F and prepare a baking sheet.
2. Combine all of the ingredients in a medium bowl and mix well to form a dough.

3. Form into a long roll and wrap tightly with plastic wrap and chill for 30 minutes then unwrap and slice into ½ inch thick rounds.
4. Bake for 12 minutes and leave to cool and firm up.
5. Melt the dark chocolate then drizzle over the shortbread and cool.

Nutrition per serving

Calories: 183

- Total Fat 14.8g
- Saturated Fat 5.3g
- Cholesterol 11mg
- Sodium 56mg
- Total Carbohydrate 14.7g
- Dietary Fiber 2.7g
- Total Sugars 0.2g
- Protein 3.9g

Chocolate Orange Cake Pops

These fun chocolate orange cake pops are perfect for parties. Try decorating with friends for a great weekend activity.

Serves: 12

Ingredients

- ⅔ cup almond butter
- ⅓ cup coconut flour
- 30 drops stevia (orange flavored)
- 6 Tbsp orange zest
- ¼ cup orange juice

For rolling

- 2 Tbsp cacao powder (sugar-free)

Method

1. Combine all the ingredients in a medium-sized bowl.
2. Divide into 12 balls and pierce with a cake pop stick. Roll in cacao powder then freeze for 20 minutes to firm up. Alternatively, stick them in the fridge overnight.

Nutrition per serving

Calories: 26

- Total Fat 1g
- Saturated Fat 0.4g
- Cholesterol 0mg
- Sodium 0mg
- Total Carbohydrate 4.1g
- Dietary Fiber 2g
- Total Sugars 0.5g
- Protein 0.9g

Red Velvet Pancakes

What more could you ever want to be served in bed on a rainy morning than these fluffy and chocolaty pancakes? Soft, sweet and delicious. Add coconut yogurt and grated coconut for extra goodness!

Serves: 12

Ingredients

- 4 eggs
- 1 cup coconut milk
- 2 Tbsp Erythritol
- 1 tsp vanilla essence
- 1 tsp red food coloring
- 1 Tbsp cocoa powder (unsweetened)
- ½ cup coconut flour
- 1 tsp baking powder
- ½ tsp sea salt
- 2 Tbsp coconut oil

Method

1. Whisk the eggs then add coconut milk and sweetener and combine well.

2. Add the vanilla, coloring, cocoa powder, coconut flour, baking powder, and salt to form a batter.
3. Heat the coconut oil in the pan on a medium heat then spoon the batter into the pan and fry until bubbles appear. Then flip the pancake and cook on the other side.
4. Serve and enjoy!

Nutrition per serving

Calories: 109

- Total Fat 9.1g
- Saturated Fat 7g
- Cholesterol 55mg
- Sodium 102mg
- Total Carbohydrate 7.6g
- Dietary Fiber 2.6g
- Total Sugars 3.3g
- Protein 3.1g

Easy Crumpets

Notoriously difficult and time-consuming to make crumpets? Not these keto friendly, 90-second breakfast treats! With just a microwave and container you can make your crumpets the night before, in less than a few minutes, and enjoy with as much butter and toppings as you wish!

Serves: 2

Ingredients

- 1 large egg
- pinch of sea salt
- 1 tsp fine coconut flour
- 1 tsp fine psyllium husk powder
- ¼ tsp baking powder
- 1 tsp flaxseed oil
- 1 tsp apple cider vinegar

Method

1. Whisk the egg until frothy and add all other ingredients, beating between each addition.
2. Grease a microwave-proof container with flaxseed oil and pour in the mixture.

3. Cook for 90 seconds and if it's still wet cook for a further 15 seconds.
4. Turn the container upside down on a cooling rack to release the steam.
5. Once cooled slice through the middle and serve toasted with butter.

Nutrition per serving

Calories: 69

- Total Fat 5g
- Saturated Fat 1.1g
- Cholesterol 93mg
- Sodium 153mg
- Total Carbohydrate 2.7g
- Dietary Fiber 1.7g
- Total Sugars 0.2g
- Protein 3.3g

Banana and Chocolate Bread

Everybody loves banana bread but add some sugar-free chocolate to the mix and you have an easy dessert or satisfying, afternoon snack. Enjoy!

Serves: 10

Ingredients

- 3 overripe banana (mashed)
- 3 large eggs
- 2 cups almond flour
- ¼ cup olive oil
- 1 tsp baking soda
- ¼ tsp sea salt
- ½ cup unsweetened dark chocolate (chopped)

Method

1. Preheat the oven to 350F and prepare a loaf pan.
2. Mix together the eggs, mashed banana, and olive oil.
3. In a separate bowl mix together the almond flour, baking soda, and sea salt.
4. Combine the two mixtures together until well blended

and add the chocolate pieces.

5. Pour in the batter and bake for 60 minutes until golden.

Nutrition per serving

Calories: 311

- Total Fat 23.7g
- Saturated Fat 6g
- Cholesterol 56mg
- Sodium 159mg
- Total Carbohydrate 16.2g
- Dietary Fiber 4.9g
- Total Sugars 4.5g
- Protein 8.7g

Beetroot Brownies

These rich and fudgy brownies literally melt in your mouth! Add nuts for an extra crunch or drizzle in nut butter.

Serves: 10

Ingredients

- 2 Tbsp flaxseed meal
- 6 Tbsp water
- 1 ¼ cup roasted beetroot
- 3 Tbsp coconut oil
- 1 ¼ cup coconut milk
- 1 Tbsp pure vanilla extract
- ¾ cup raw cacao powder
- ¼ cup tapioca starch*
- ¾ cup coconut sugar
- 1 ¼ cups almond flour
- 1 ½ teaspoons baking powder
- ¼ tsp baking soda
- ½ tsp sea salt
- ¼ tsp ground cinnamon

Method

1. Preheat the oven to 375F and prepare a baking dish.
2. Mix together the water and flax meal and leave to thicken for about 10 minutes, stirring occasionally.
3. Add the roasted beetroot to a blender and blend for a few seconds to a smooth puree.
4. Add the flax mixture and the remaining ingredients to the blender. Blend very well until completely smooth.
5. Pour the brownie batter into the prepared baking dish and bake for 45 to 55 minutes and allow to cool for 30 minutes before cutting into pieces.

Nutrition per serving

Calories: 312

- Total Fat 19.3g
- Saturated Fat 10.8g
- Cholesterol 0mg
- Sodium 158mg
- Total Carbohydrate 30g
- Dietary Fiber 6.1g
- Total Sugars 17g
- Protein 5.6g

Parmesan Croutons

Make texture free salads a thing of the past with these crunchy keto croutons, give a bite to your soup or take a small bag to work as a mid-morning snack just as they are.

Serves: 6

Ingredients

- ½ cup almond flour
- 4 tsp psyllium husk fiber
- 1 tsp baking powder
- 1 tsp garlic powder
- ¼ tsp salt
- ¼ tsp cracked black pepper
- 2 egg whites
- 1 Tbsp coconut oil
- 2 Tbsp Parmesan cheese (grated)

Method

1. Heat oven to 350F and prepare a baking sheet.
2. Combine almond flour, psyllium fiber, baking powder, garlic and salt in a large bowl.

3. Mix in the egg whites until you have a sticky dough mix

4. Roll out the dough on your baking sheet until even, then bake for 10 minutes until it starts to firm up.

5. Remove from the oven and cut the dough into small crouton pieces. Drizzle with oil and Parmesan then return to oven until golden brown. Leave to cool for extra crunch!

Nutrition per serving

Calories: 89

- Total Fat 7.1g
- Saturated Fat 2.5g
- Cholesterol 1mg
- Sodium 128mg
- Total Carbohydrate 4.6g
- Dietary Fiber 2.8g
- Total Sugars 0.2g
- Protein 3.8g

Avocado Chocolate Cake

It's not how it sounds, and it's definitely not green! The avocado in this cake creates a rich and fudgy texture whilst the coconut cream gives a fresh and tangy flavor to every bite of chocolate heaven.

Serves: 12

Ingredients

Sponge

- 2 cups almond flour
- ½ cup cocoa powder (sugar-free)
- ½ cup monk fruit sweetener
- 1 tsp baking soda
- ¼ tsp sea salt
- 1 avocado
- ½ cup coconut yogurt
- ½ cup almond milk
- 2 eggs

Frosting

- ½ avocado
- 2 Tbsp coconut cream
- 2 Tbsp vanilla

- 2 Tbsp coconut oil (melted)
- 2 Tbsp cocoa powder (sugar-free)

Method

1. Preheat oven to 350F, and prepare a baking pan.
2. Mix together all the dry ingredients in one bowl and the wet ingredients in another.
3. When both mixes are thoroughly combined and there's no noticeable avocado you can fold the dry mix into the wet to form the batter.
4. Pour into the pan and bake for 30 - 40 minutes.
5. Whilst the cake cools, create the frosting by combining all the ingredients and blending until smooth.
6. Pipe the frosting onto your cooled sponge and serve!

Nutrition per serving

Calories: 241

- Total Fat 19.8g
- Saturated Fat 6.6g
- Cholesterol 27mg
- Sodium 164mg
- Total Carbohydrate 18.2g
- Dietary Fiber 3.9g

- Total Sugars 3.1g
- Protein 6.2g

Courgette, Lemon & Mascarpone Cupcakes

Bursting with zingy lemons, green-powered courgette, and creamy, fresh mascarpone.

Serves: 8

Ingredients

Sponge

- 6 medium eggs
- ¾ cup coconut flour
- 1 cup zucchini (grated)
- ⅓ cup coconut oil (melted)
- ¼ cup stevia
- ½ tsp baking soda
- 4 tsp lemon zest

Frosting

- 1 cup mascarpone cheese
- ¼ cup powdered erythritol
- ¼ cup heavy cream
- 2 tsp fresh lemon juice
- 2 tsp lemon zest
- 1 tsp vanilla

Method

1. Preheat the oven to 355F and prepare a muffin pan with paper cups.
2. Mix together all the ingredients until well combined.
3. Fill each cup with batter and bake for 25 minutes, remove to cool on a wire tray.
4. Whilst the cakes cool, whip the mascarpone until light and fluffy.
5. Add the remaining ingredients then mix until smooth.
6. Pipe the frosting onto the cupcakes and sprinkle with lemon zest.

Nutrition per serving

Calories: 250

- Total Fat 18.9g
- Saturated Fat 13.1g
- Cholesterol 144mg
- Sodium 155mg
- Total Carbohydrate 14.2g
- Dietary Fiber 4.8g
- Total Sugars 0.8g
- Protein 9.4g

Sourdough

Everybody loves this famously fermented superfood and now you can impress your friends and make your own! The perfect accompaniment to avo on toast.

Serves: 8

Ingredients

- 1 ½ cup almond flour
- ⅓ cup psyllium husk powder
- ½ cup coconut flour
- ½ cup flax meal
- 1 tsp salt baking soda
- 1 tsp sea salt
- 6 large egg whites
- 2 large eggs
- ¾ cup buttermilk
- ¼ cup apple cider vinegar
- ½ cup lukewarm water

Method

1. Preheat the oven to 360F and prepare a baking sheet.
2. Mix all the dry ingredients together in one bowl.

3. Next, add the eggs, egg whites, and buttermilk in a separate mixing bowl and combine. Add both the mixes together then add vinegar and lukewarm water and process until well combined.
4. Shape as desired and place in the oven and bake for 35-40 minutes remove and place on a cooling rack until it reaches room temperature.

Nutrition per serving

Calories: 222

- Total Fat 12.5g
- Saturated Fat 1.8g
- Cholesterol 47mg
- Sodium 468mg
- Total Carbohydrate 16.6g
- Dietary Fiber 10.2g
- Total Sugars 1.4g
- Protein 10.7g

Peanut Butter Cookies

Only five ingredients needed, these super easy peanut butter cookies are easy to make, easier to eat and irresistible for late night cravings.

Serves: 10

Ingredients

- ½ cup peanut butter
- ½ cup powdered erythritol
- 1 egg
- 1 tsp vanilla
- ¼ tsp sea salt

Method

1. Preheat oven to 350F and prepare a baking sheet.
2. Simply mix together all the ingredients in a large bowl until a dough is formed.
3. Split the mixture into even balls, roll and flatten slightly with your thumb before placing on the baking tray.
4. Bake for 12-15 minutes and cool for 10!

Nutrition per serving

Calories: 96

- Total Fat 6.9g
- Saturated Fat 1.5g
- Cholesterol 16mg
- Sodium 112mg
- Total Carbohydrate 9.8g
- Dietary Fiber 0.8g
- Total Sugars 1.3g
- Protein 3.8g

Pretzels

A German delicacy which goes far too well with a Bavarian beer, this ideal finger food is the perfect easy snack for movie nights and football games.

Serves: 12

Ingredients

- 3 cups mozzarella cheese (shredded)
- 4 Tbsp of cream cheese
- 2 tsp of dried yeast
- 2 Tbsp of warm water
- 1 ½ cups of almond flour
- 2 tsp of xanthan gum
- 2 eggs
- 2 Tbsp butter (melted)
- 1 Tbsp sea salt

Method

1. Preheat oven to 390F and prepare a baking sheet.
2. Mix the cheese together and microwave for 30 seconds at a time, stirring in between each installment, until fully melted.

3. Activate the yeast by dissolving it in the warm water and leaving for 2 minutes.
4. Combine the almond flour and xanthum gum and add in the eggs, yeast mix, butter and cheese until well combined. Knead for 10 minutes.
5. Divide the dough into 12 balls and roll them into even, thin 'sausage' shapes. Twist into a pretzel shape and brush with a little egg or milk, then sprinkle with sea salt.
6. Bake in the oven for 12-15 minutes until golden brown.

Nutrition per serving

Calories: 145

- Total Fat 11.7g
- Saturated Fat 3.4g
- Cholesterol 40mg
- Sodium 132mg
- Total Carbohydrate 4g
- Dietary Fiber 2g
- Total Sugars 0.1g
- Protein 6.5g

Coconut Macaroons

French, fabulous macaroons full of almond, coconut, chocolate goodness. These look so much more time consuming than the reality and taste as good as the classic. Enjoy!

Serves: 12

Ingredients

- 2 egg whites
- ⅓ cup erythritol sweetener
- 1 tsp almond extract
- ¼ tsp sea salt
- 2 cups unsweetened shredded coconut
- 2 oz dark chocolate chips (sugar-free)

Method

1. Preheat the oven to 325F and prepare a baking sheet.
2. Whisk the egg whites until medium - stiff peaks start to form.
3. Add in 1 spoonful of sweetener at a time, whilst constantly whisking. Then gradually add in the salt, almond and coconut flakes.

4. Spoon the mix onto the baking sheet and bake for 15 to 20 minutes, until golden brown.
5. When the macaroons are cooled, melt the chocolate and dip the macaroons so the base is covered, cool and enjoy!

Nutrition per serving

Calories: 146

- Total Fat 11.9g
- Saturated Fat 10.1g
- Cholesterol 0mg
- Sodium 51mg
- Total Carbohydrate 7.2g
- Dietary Fiber 2.7g
- Total Sugars 3.9g
- Protein 2.2g

Cumin Naan

Aromatic cumin and oozing in buttery parsley. Warm, crispy and delicious.

Serves: 8

Ingredients

- ¾ cup coconut flour
- 2 Tbsp ground psyllium husk powder
- ½ tsp onion powder
- ½ tsp garlic granules
- ½ tsp baking powder
- 1/3 cup coconut oil (melted)
- 2 cups boiling water
- ½ tsp sea salt
- 1 Tbsp cumin

Topping

- 2 Tbsp butter (melted)
- 2 Tbsp parsley (chopped)

Method

1. Combine all the dry ingredients in a medium bowl then add oil and boiling water and stir well. Leave to prove for five minutes.
2. Divide into 8 even pieces and roll into balls then flatten with your hands directly onto a floured surface.
3. Grease a skillet to stop the naan bread sticking, then fry the dough on a medium heat.
4. Mix the butter and parsley together and brush over the warm naan bread using a pastry brush.

Nutrition per serving

Calories: 160

- Total Fat 13.3g
- Saturated Fat 10.4g
- Cholesterol 8mg
- Sodium 141mg
- Total Carbohydrate 10.2g
- Dietary Fiber 6.4g
- Total Sugars 0.1g
- Protein 1.7g

Carrot Cake Cookies

Carrot cake IN a cookie, enough said! Have your favorite dessert on the go and nibble away all day long on these crispy carrot goodies.

Serves: 12

Ingredients

- ¾ cup almond flour
- ¼ cup coconut flour
- 1 large egg
- 4 Tbsp butter
- ¾ cup erythritol
- ¼ tsp baking soda
- ¼ tsp sea salt
- ⅓ cup walnuts (chopped)
- ¼ cup shredded carrots (chopped)

Method

1. Preheat your oven to 350F and prepare a baking sheet.
2. Mix together the flours, baking soda, and salt in one bowl.

3. Melt the butter in a separate mixing bowl and add the erythritol and eggs.
4. Combine the two mixes and add the walnuts and carrots to form the batter.
5. Separate into even balls, roll and flatten as preferred and place onto a baking sheet.
6. Bake for 12-14 minutes then allow to cool for 15 minutes.

Nutrition per serving

Calories: 115

- Total Fat 9.9g
- Saturated Fat 3.1g
- Cholesterol 26mg
- Sodium 69mg
- Total Carbohydrate 19.2g
- Dietary Fiber 2.1g
- Total Sugars 15.2g
- Protein 3.2g

Chocolate Pizza

The pizza party doesn't have to end when dinner does, now you can have your favorite meal for dessert, too! Have fun customizing the toppings and using up whatever you have in the cupboard.

Serves: 10

Ingredients

Pizza base

- 2 cups almond flour
- ⅓ cup cacao powder
- ¼ sea salt
- 6 Tbsp coconut oil (melted)
- 5 Tbsp almond milk
- 2 Tbsp ground flaxseed
- 3 tsp vanilla
- ½ cup chocolate pieces (sugar-free)

Sauce

- ¾ cup chocolate pieces (sugar-free)
- 2 Tbsp avocado oil

Toppings

- ½ cup raspberries
- ½ cup strawberries
- 2 Tbsp hazelnuts
- 2 Tbsp rainbow sprinkles (sugar-free)

Method

1. Preheat oven to 375F and prepare a pizza dish.
2. Mix together the flour, cacao and salt.
3. In a separate bowl, stir together flax and milk and let sit for 5 minutes to thicken. Whisk together remaining wet ingredients and pour over the flour mixture. Stir well then add the chocolate.
4. Roll out the dough onto the pan and fill the dish like you would with a savory pizza. Bake for 10 -12 min and leave to cool and firm up.
5. Melt your second bowl of chocolate and stir in the oil until smooth.
6. Spread the sauce over the base, leaving a ½ inch border for the crust.
7. Sprinkle your toppings on and slice into 'pizza' slices!

Nutrition per serving

Calories: 360

- Total Fat 25.5g
- Saturated Fat 7.8g
- Cholesterol 5mg
- Sodium 230mg
- Total Carbohydrate 25.2g
- Dietary Fiber 5g
- Total Sugars 14.7g
- Protein 8g

Spicy Cheese Taco Shells

These spicy tacos are a tangy and crisp keto alternative packing even more Mexican flavor than the classic. Fill with ground beef, roasted veg or your favorite salad - just don't forget the tequila!

Serves: 8

Ingredients

- 2 cup Mexican cheese (shredded)
- ½ Tbsp paprika
- ¼ tsp red chili flakes

Method

1. Preheat oven to 350F and prepare a baking sheet.
2. In a bowl mix all the ingredients together. Spread out ⅛ of the cheese mix into a circle, large enough for one taco.
3. Bake for 8 minutes until bubbling and going slightly golden.
4. When it's just cool enough to touch, bend it into your taco shape using a glass as a mold. Leave for 2-3 minutes to firm up then add fillings and enjoy.

Nutrition per serving

Calories: 113

- Total Fat 10.1g
- Saturated Fat 5.6g
- Cholesterol 28mg
- Sodium 212mg
- Total Carbohydrate 1.4g
- Dietary Fiber 0.2g
- Total Sugars 0.1g
- Protein 6.8g

Conclusion

This recipe book might go against the grain when it comes to keto baking and you'll no doubt be surprised by the amount of 'naughty' food we have included. However, every single recipe in the book has been created for you, it won't break the food plan and it might be more decadent and delicious than you ever thought a keto diet could be.

www.ingramcontent.com/pod-product-compliance
Lightning Source LLC
Chambersburg PA
CBHW071357080526
44587CB00017B/3116